P9-BIU-861

101
ESSENTIAL TIPS

CHILDBIRTH

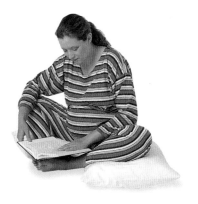

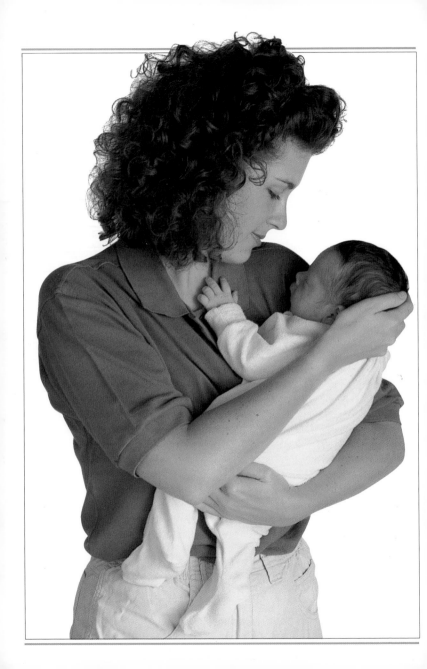

ESSENTIAL TIPS

101

CHILDBIRTH

Elizabeth Fenwick

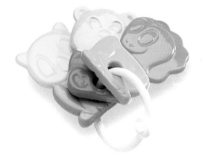

DK PUBLISHING, INC.

www.dk.com

LONDON, NEW YORK, MUNICH,
MELBOURNE, AND DELHI

Editor James Harrison
Art Editor Sharon Rudd
Series Editor Charlotte Davies
Series Art Editor Clive Hayball
Production Controller Lauren Britton
US Editor Laaren Brown

First American Edition, 1996
2 4 6 8 10 9 7 5 3
Published in the United States by DK Publishing, Inc.
375 Hudson Street
New York, New York 10014

see our complete product line at
www.dk.com

Copyright © 1996 Dorling Kindersley Limited, London

All rights reserved under International and Pan-American Copyright Conventions. No part
of this publication may be reproduced, stored in a retrieval system, or transmitted in any
form or by any means, electronic, mechanical, photocopying, recording or otherwise,
without the prior written permission of the copyright owner.
Published in Great Britain by Dorling Kindersley Limited.

ISBN 0–7894–1079–6

Text film output by The Right Type, Great Britain
Reproduced by Colourscan, Singapore
Printed in Hong Kong by Wing King Tong

ESSENTIAL TIPS

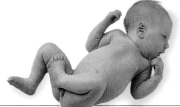

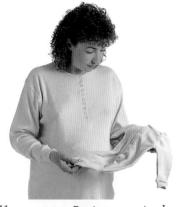

FIRST STAGES OF LABOR

OPTIONS FOR BIRTH

PAIN RELIEF

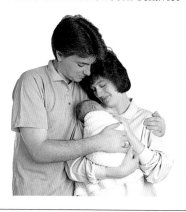

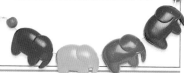

BECOMING PREGNANT

1 FIRST SIGNS OF PREGNANCY

The obvious signs are enlarged, tender breasts, which perhaps tingle a little, and feeling sick at any time of the day. You may also have a strange metallic taste in your mouth and feel a frequent need to urinate. Missing a period does not, in itself, mean you are pregnant, especially if your periods are irregular or you are anxious or ill. But check it against the other signs.

2 CONFIRMING THE PREGNANCY

Have the pregnancy confirmed as soon as possible. There are a variety of professional and do-it-yourself tests available – the most accurate are provided by your doctor or family planning clinic. A urine sample taken about two weeks after your first missed period will detect a hormone that confirms the pregnancy.

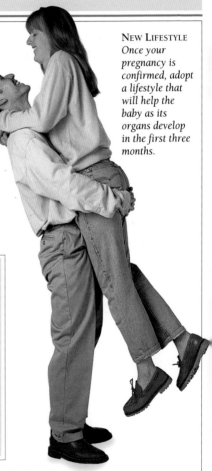

NEW LIFESTYLE
Once your pregnancy is confirmed, adopt a lifestyle that will help the baby as its organs develop in the first three months.

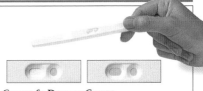

3 HOME PREGNANCY TESTS

Home pregnancy test kits use a chemical solution which you mix with a urine sample. A color change will detect the hormone made by the embryo (called HCG), which confirms the pregnancy.

CHECK & DOUBLE-CHECK
Home tests are fairly accurate and usually a reliable guide. But you should still confirm a pregnancy with your doctor.

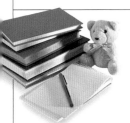

4 CALCULATE YOUR DUE DATE

From conception you will be pregnant for some 266 days. Conception usually occurs when you ovulate, that is, about 14 days before your next period. To work out the date of birth, count 280 days (266 + 14) from the first day of your last period.

Find the first day of your last period on the top line; the line underneath is the due date

January Oct/Nov	1 2 3 4 5 6 7 8 9 10 11 12 13 14 15 16 17 18 19 20 21 22 23 24 25 26 27 28 29 30 31
	8 9 10 11 12 13 14 15 16 17 18 19 20 21 22 23 24 25 26 27 28 29 30 31 1 2 3 4 5 6 7
February Nov/Dec	1 2 3 4 5 6 7 8 9 10 11 12 13 14 15 16 17 18 19 20 21 22 23 24 25 26 27 28
	8 9 10 11 12 13 14 15 16 17 18 19 20 21 22 23 24 25 26 27 28 29 30 1 2 3 4 5
March Dec/Jan	1 2 3 4 5 6 7 8 9 10 11 12 13 14 15 16 17 18 19 20 21 22 23 24 25 26 27 28 29 30 31
	6 7 8 9 10 11 12 13 14 15 16 17 18 19 20 21 22 23 24 25 26 27 28 29 30 31 1 2 3 4 5
April Jan/Feb	1 2 3 4 5 6 7 8 9 10 11 12 13 14 15 16 17 18 19 20 21 22 23 24 25 26 27 28 29 30
	6 7 8 9 10 11 12 13 14 15 16 17 18 19 20 21 22 23 24 25 26 27 28 29 30 31 1 2 3 4
May Feb/March	1 2 3 4 5 6 7 8 9 10 11 12 13 14 15 16 17 18 19 20 21 22 23 24 25 26 27 28 29 30 31
	5 6 7 8 9 10 11 12 13 14 15 16 17 18 19 20 21 22 23 24 25 26 27 28 1 2 3 4 5 6 7
June March/April	1 2 3 4 5 6 7 8 9 10 11 12 13 14 15 16 17 18 19 20 21 22 23 24 25 26 27 28 29 30
	8 9 10 11 12 13 14 15 16 17 18 19 20 21 22 23 24 25 26 27 28 29 30 31 1 2 3 4 5 6
July April/May	1 2 3 4 5 6 7 8 9 10 11 12 13 14 15 16 17 18 19 20 21 22 23 24 25 26 27 28 29 30 31
	7 8 9 10 11 12 13 14 15 16 17 18 19 20 21 22 23 24 25 26 27 28 29 30 1 2 3 4 5 6 7
August May/June	1 2 3 4 5 6 7 8 9 10 11 12 13 14 15 16 17 18 19 20 21 22 23 24 25 26 27 28 29 30 31
	8 9 10 11 12 13 14 15 16 17 18 19 20 21 22 23 24 25 26 27 28 29 30 31 1 2 3 4 5 6 7
September June/July	1 2 3 4 5 6 7 8 9 10 11 12 13 14 15 16 17 18 19 20 21 22 23 24 25 26 27 28 29 30
	8 9 10 11 12 13 14 15 16 17 18 19 20 21 22 23 24 25 26 27 28 29 30 1 2 3 4 5 6 7
October July/August	1 2 3 4 5 6 7 8 9 10 11 12 13 14 15 16 17 18 19 20 21 22 23 24 25 26 27 28 29 30 31
	8 9 10 11 12 13 14 15 16 17 18 19 20 21 22 23 24 25 26 27 28 29 30 31 1 2 3 4 5 6 7
November August/Sept	1 2 3 4 5 6 7 8 9 10 11 12 13 14 15 16 17 18 19 20 21 22 23 24 25 26 27 28 29 30
	8 9 10 11 12 13 14 15 16 17 18 19 20 21 22 23 24 25 26 27 28 29 30 31 1 2 3 4 5 6
December Sept/Oct	1 2 3 4 5 6 7 8 9 10 11 12 13 14 15 16 17 18 19 20 21 22 23 24 25 26 27 28 29 30 31
	7 8 9 10 11 12 13 14 15 16 17 18 19 20 21 22 23 24 25 26 27 28 29 30 1 2 3 4 5 6 7

5 YOUR PREGNANCY CALENDAR

Nine months and two weeks is the average pregnancy, but this can vary by as much as a month. The changes your body undergo fall into roughly three three-month stages (called trimesters), and these can be broken down into four-week periods as a yardstick to judge what should be happening to you. Remember, every mother

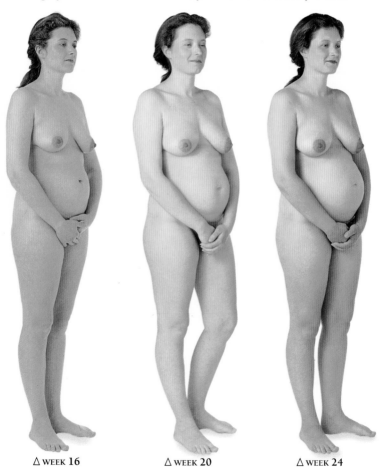

△ WEEK 16   △ WEEK 20   △ WEEK 24

is different, so pregnancy weight gains and fetus length and weight gains will vary. Emotionally it can be both a very positive and a very anxious time. Fetal abnormalities most often occur in the first few weeks after conception, so it is important to take care of yourself even if you are not anticipating becoming pregnant. By week 13, when your baby is fully formed, very little can go wrong.

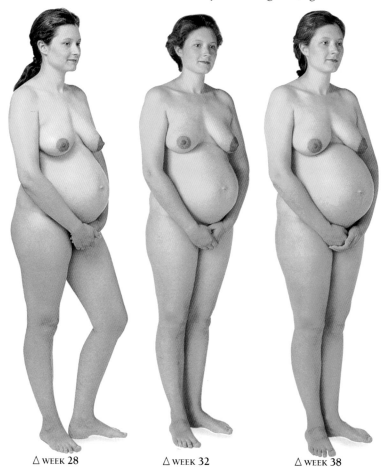

△ WEEK 28   △ WEEK 32   △ WEEK 38

VISITING THE DOCTOR

6 YOUR FIRST VISIT

This should take place about 12 weeks after you confirm your pregnancy. The doctor or midwife will check on the personal details of you and your partner. They will also ask about your family medical history: for instance, if twins run in the family, as well as about what form of contraceptives you used, when your periods began, and when the first day of your last period was. You will also be asked about previous pregnancies.

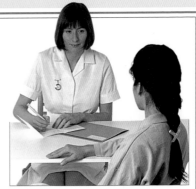

FIRST VISIT
This sets the scene for all your visits to come. You should be going once a month after your first visit up to week 28.

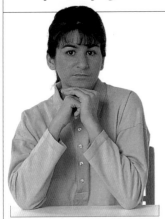

7 ASKING QUESTIONS

After your doctor has asked you questions, you should be prepared with any questions you have, for instance:
- which pain relief is available;
- who can be present at the labor;
- what positions you can give birth in;
- whether chairs, large cushions, or birthing stools are available.

QUESTION TO ASK
Have a "shopping list" of questions ready and ask for clarification if you don't understand the answers. Everything should be explained fully and simply.

8 CHECKING HEIGHT & WEIGHT

At your first visit your height and weight will be measured. You will also be weighed to check whether you are over- or underweight. Your starting weight is also needed to check whether you are gaining weight properly as the pregnancy progresses. Try to wear similar clothes for each visit. Don't worry if you lose weight in the first three months from morning sickness.

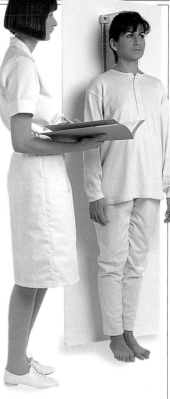

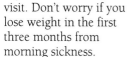

◁△ LOOKING FOR AVERAGES
Checking your weight gain, along with your height, plus blood and urine tests, sonograms, and other tests, gives a reliable guide to the rate of the baby's growth.

MEASURING YOUR HEIGHT
Checking your height can help to indicate potential problems if you are very short in comparison to the average height for your racial and/or ethnic type and build.

13

9 BLOOD TESTS (& RH FACTOR)

Some blood will be taken from your arm to check the following:
- That you are not anemic (lacking iron). During pregnancy your blood volume increases and the baby takes iron from you to form its own blood. Thus your stores of iron can easily become depleted at this time.
- That you are immune to German measles, which can cause serious defects. (This should ideally have been checked before pregnancy.)
- That you do not have a sexually transmitted disease. If you do have an STD, discuss it with your doctor as soon as possible.

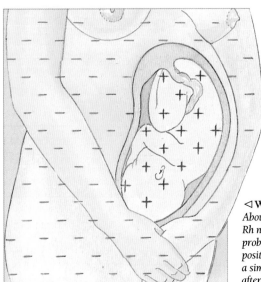

THE RH FACTOR
A key part of a blood test is to check your blood group and see if you are an "Rh negative" mother carrying an "Rh positive baby" – a problem that can be safeguarded against.

◁ WHAT RH NEGATIVE MEANS
About 15 percent of mothers are Rh negative which is only a problem if they have an Rh positive baby. Treatment involves a simple protective vaccination after the first pregnancy.

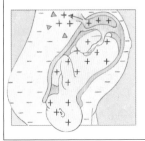

◁ FIRST BABY
The blood of the Rh+ baby in an Rh- mother's bloodstream can destroy red blood cells.

SECOND BABY ▷
Special blood injections protect the second baby.

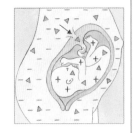

10 BLOOD PRESSURE

Normal blood pressure is around 120/70. During pregnancy it will be slightly lower. It will be measured at each visit to check that it does not rise above 140/90. Raised blood pressure can be a sign of several problems, including preeclampsia (*see p.23*).

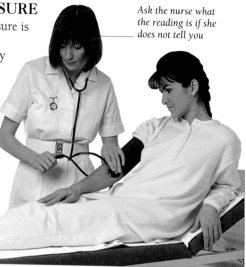

Ask the nurse what the reading is if she does not tell you

KEEP THE PRESSURE DOWN ▷
Anxiety and waiting for tests can cause a higher reading than normal. If so, your blood pressure can be taken again.

11 URINE TESTS

Take a sample of first morning urine with you to each visit. This will be tested for:
- traces of sugar, which, if detected repeatedly, could be a sign of diabetes (*see p.22*);
- traces of protein, which could be a sign that your kidneys are not functioning properly. Protein found later in pregnancy could also indicate preeclampsia (*see p.23*).

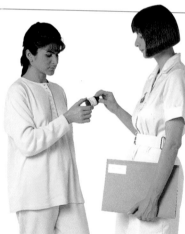

MIDSTREAM URINE SAMPLE
Urinate in the toilet first, then collect a sample of the midstream drops in the sterile container.

INSTANT CHECK
On a first visit you will be given a sterile swab of cotton to wipe yourself clean and a sterile container to urinate into. The urine is tested immediately.

12 LEGS, ANKLES, & HANDS

The doctor or midwife will inspect your lower legs, ankles, and hands, and feel them to confirm there is no swelling or puffiness (known as edema). If the veins in your calves and thighs become painful and swollen and you have aching legs, this may mean you have varicose veins. A check will be made for this.

Some swelling of the wrists is normal near the end of pregnancy

◁ **CHECK SWELLINGS**
Excessive swelling of the ankles or wrists may be a sign of preeclampsia (see p.23). A little swelling, especially at the end of the day, in the last few weeks is normal.

Ankles felt for signs of edema

13 FEELING THE ABDOMEN

The doctor will feel your abdomen gently to check the position of the top of the uterus. This gives an indication of the rate of the baby's growth. Later on, checks will be made to ensure that your baby is turning the right way around (head first) and, in the final weeks, that the head is dropping into the pelvis (known as engaging).

UTERUS CHECK
The top of your uterus (fundus) will also be felt and the distance measured between that and the pelvic bone to check the baby's rate of growth between visits.

EXTERNAL PALPITATIONS ▷
By feeling your abdomen at each visit the doctor can build an accurate picture of your baby's rate of progress against its due date.

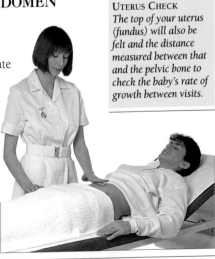

14 INTERNAL EXAMINATION

Not every woman has an internal examination at the first visit, but a doctor may decide on one to confirm the pregnancy and to check that the cervix entrance to the uterus is tightly closed. A Pap smear may be taken to test for abnormal (precancerous) cells. The internal examination will not hurt you or your baby, so there is no need to be worried about this part of the visit. All these tests are carried out in order to ensure a healthy pregnancy.

FIRST EXAMINATION ▽
On your first examination the doctor or midwife will listen to your heart and lungs and examine your breasts to check for lumps and for inverted or flat nipples (with a view to breast-feeding).

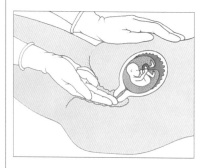

◁ CHECKING THE UTERUS
The doctor will insert two gloved fingers of one hand into the vagina and press your abdomen gently with the other hand. Other internal checks include checking the "passageway" size for delivery.

15 MORNING SICKNESS

This is one of the first signs of being pregnant, but it can occur at any time of the day. If you are tired, your nausea may be worse. It often comes on when you haven't eaten for a while, hence "morning" sickness. Nausea is often heightened by the smell of cigarettes or certain foods. In many cases, nausea lasts for 12 weeks, then disappears. However, it can return later in the pregnancy. Obviously, try to avoid those smells and foods that make you feel sick. Eat foods that appeal to you to keep nausea at bay and try eating small, frequent meals.

16 LISTEN TO YOUR BABY'S HEARTBEAT

After week 14 your baby's heartbeat may be checked with an electronic "sonicaid," a small listening device, which is placed on your stomach and uses ultrasound to amplify the fetal heartbeat so that you can hear it, too. Occasionally, an old-fashioned trumpet-shaped fetal stethoscope may be used to monitor the heartbeat after week 28. A baby's heart rate, at 140 beats per minute, is double that of an adult, at roughly 72 beats a minute.

17 HOW YOUR BABY LIES

At your first prenatal visit, your doctor or midwife will begin your file, recording the medical details of your pregnancy in abbreviated form. It details all the routine tests, and charts the progress that you make at each visit. Among the various abbreviations are those used by doctors, midwives, and nurses to describe the way the baby is lying in the uterus. They relate to the position of the back of the baby's head (occiput) in relation to your body. The key abbreviations are given here.

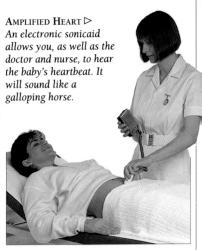

AMPLIFIED HEART ▷
An electronic sonicaid allows you, as well as the doctor and nurse, to hear the baby's heartbeat. It will sound like a galloping horse.

SIMPLE STETHOSCOPE ▷
A fetal stethoscope is an easy way for the doctor to listen to the baby's heartbeat.

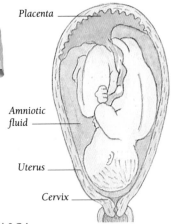

Placenta

Amniotic fluid

Uterus

Cervix

△ LOA
O=Occiput (back of a baby's head), L=Left, A=Anterior (pointing forward). Occiput faces forward on left of mother's uterus.

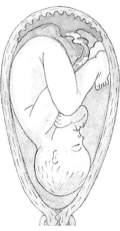

△ **ROL**
The back of the baby's head is lying to the right side on your right.

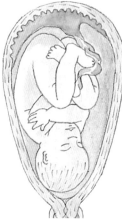

△ **ROP**
The back of the baby's head is lying to the back on your right.

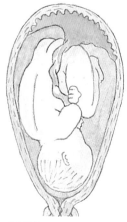

△ **ROA**
The back of the baby's head is lying to the front on your right.

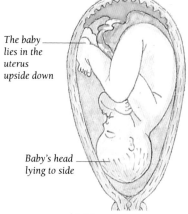

The baby lies in the uterus upside down

Baby's head lying to side

△ **LOL**
The back of the baby's head is lying to the left side on your left.

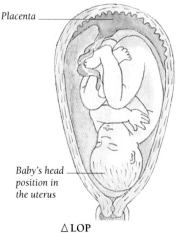

Placenta

Baby's head position in the uterus

△ **LOP**
The back of the baby's head is lying to the back on the left of your uterus.

EXTRA TESTS & SPECIAL CARE

18 SONOGRAMS

A sonogram, or ultrasound scan, is a routine part of checking a baby's progress, but is also given to check the following:

- infertility problems
- certain abdominal problems
- suspected imminent miscarriage
- suspected multiple pregnancy.

The routine check normally comes at week 16. Since this is the first time you "see" your baby (on screen) it is exciting and worth sharing with your partner. The sonogram may reveal your baby's sex; tell the technician and doctor in advance if you do not want to know.

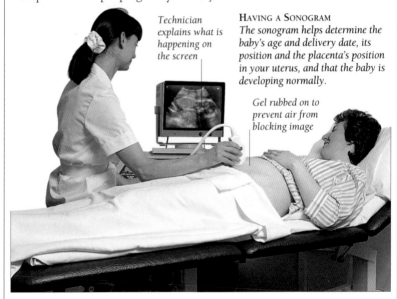

Technician explains what is happening on the screen

HAVING A SONOGRAM
The sonogram helps determine the baby's age and delivery date, its position and the placenta's position in your uterus, and that the baby is developing normally.

Gel rubbed on to prevent air from blocking image

19 SCREENING FOR ABNORMALITIES

Certain tests are offered for suspected abnormalities such as Down syndrome (mongolism). The tests are carried out on cells from the unborn baby that are obtained by amniocentesis *(see p.23)* or chorionic villi sampling. The cells are allowed to grow and divide, and are then examined to see whether they contain the right number of chromosomes (23 pairs). Sometimes it is important to know the sex of the baby, too, as certain disorders are sex-linked.

Abnormalities What are they?	Pregnancies at risk	Screening procedure	What can be done
Developmental abnormalities These are disorders occurring after fertilization, such as spina bifida	Small risk in pregnancies. Cause may be due to exposure to certain toxins or to a lack of folic acid	A sonogram and/or amniocentesis *(see p.23)*; or a serum screening/blood test may detect some types	Some of these defects can be prevented by good nutrition and vaccination before you get pregnant
Chromosome abnormalities Damage occurs to the chromosome as the egg or sperm develops; Down syndrome is one example of this	There is increased risk if the mother is over 35 or if the father is elderly. Even when both parents are under 35 it may occur spontaneously	Chromosome analysis on fetal cells is obtained by amniocentesis, chorionic villi sampling (similar in procedure), or fetal blood sampling	No specific treatment exists at present: the parents' chromosomes should be checked before any future pregnancy
Genetic defects Disorders like hemophilia are caused by individual gene defects. The damaged gene is then passed on to the next generation	Almost no risk if there is no family history of these disorders. However, certain genetic conditions are more prevalent in specific ethnic groups	Again, during early pregnancy amniocentesis *(see p.23)* or chorionic villi sampling can reveal a few of these gene disorders but not all	Tests are now available for some of these genetic disorders; they can determine whether or not prospective parents carry these faulty genes

20 DIABETES

This condition makes the body unable to absorb glucose, which then builds up in the blood. If you are diabetic, then your blood sugar level must be constantly monitored and kept stable. Your doctor will adjust your insulin intake and advise you about diet. You will need more prenatal visits, too, but provided these precautions are taken, your pregnancy should go smoothly. Some women suffer from a mild form of diabetes for the first time during pregnancy. Fortunately this condition nearly always disappears soon after the the birth of the baby.

21 ANEMIA

Many women are slightly anemic before pregnancy due to iron deficiency. You will need to correct the increased demand for iron to cope with pregnancy. Eat plenty of iron-rich foods such as spinach and red meat (but avoid liver products). Take iron supplement tablets after meals with a fluid.

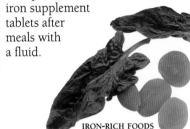

IRON-RICH FOODS

22 INCOMPETENT CERVIX

The cervix (neck of the uterus) stays closed until labor starts in a normal pregnancy. If the neck is "incompetent," or weak, then it can open up and expel the baby. This is often the reason for miscarriages occurring after the third month. Treatment is usually a small operation to stitch the cervix firmly closed.

STITCHING A WEAK CERVIX ▷
At the beginning of pregnancy, a suture, like the strings of a purse, is stitched around the cervix. The thread is cut at the end of pregnancy or as labor starts.

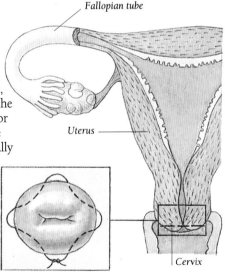

Fallopian tube

Uterus

Cervix

23 PREECLAMPSIA

This is a common problem in late pregnancy. Its most obvious warning sign is elevated blood pressure. Other symptoms are excessive weight gain; swollen ankles, feet, or hands; and traces of protein in the urine. The best course of action is to get plenty of rest, which your doctor will advise, as well as cutting down on the amount of salt you eat. You might also be given a drug to lower blood pressure.

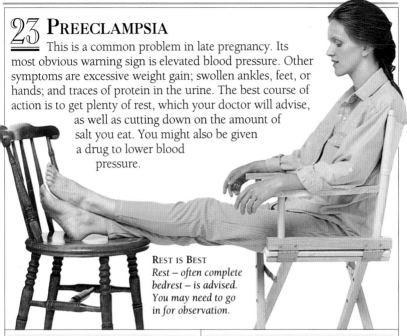

REST IS BEST
Rest – often complete bedrest – is advised. You may need to go in for observation.

24 MISCARRIAGE

A miscarriage is the ending of a pregnancy before 28 weeks, usually because the baby is not developing normally. As many as one in five pregnancies terminate this way. Many occur in the first five weeks, often before the woman knows she is pregnant. The first sign is bleeding from the vagina, but if you lie down and call the doctor immediately and bleeding is mild and painless, the pregnancy can often be saved. All vaginal bleeding should be reported to your doctor or midwife immediately.

25 AMNIOCENTESIS

If you are over 35, have a family history of inherited disease (such as spina bifida), or raised AFP (alpha-fetoprotein) levels in your blood, you may be offered an amniocentesis to aid diagnosis of possible fetal disorders. In an "amnig" a hollow needle is inserted through the wall of the stomach into the womb, and a sample of the amniotic fluid that surrounds the baby is taken. Results can take seven days, and about one in 100 tests may result in a miscarriage.

PRACTICAL PREPARATIONS

26 THINKING ABOUT CLASSES

Childbirth classes help prepare you and your partner for the practicalities of a healthy pregnancy, labor, childbirth, and essential baby care. They are a worthwhile experience, especially for first-time parents, and an excellent way to share concerns, problems, and advice. The network of mothers-to-be that classes create can be a great "extended family" support.

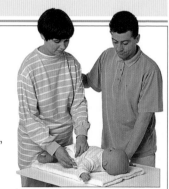

BASICS OF BABY CARE ARE TAUGHT

27 BIRTH PLANS

A birth plan is simply a written instruction sheet outlining the kind of birth you would like and noting all the issues that are important to you. Discuss these with your doctor, midwife, and prenatal class teacher, and find out what is possible at your hospital. Your plan should be feasible in terms of hospital practices, but don't be intimidated if hospital staff appear unreasonably negative. Involve your partner in your decision-making to build a sharing atmosphere for the birth.

28 MAKING YOUR OWN BIRTH PLAN

Explore all the options that you consider to be important, and after discussing them, type out your plan in a letter or list format, and sign it. Give it to your doctor at least one month before delivery. List special dietary needs, who your birthing assistant is, and if you want that person present in the delivery room. You can also include preferences about pain relief and fetal monitoring, whether you intend to breast-feed, and if you want your pubic hair shaved.

29 UNDERSTANDING BREAST-FEEDING

Your prenatal classes will advise you on the practicalities of breast-feeding and you can listen to the advice and comments of other mothers and professionals, weigh the pros and cons, and decide how this is going to fit in with your lifestyle and feelings. Even if you prefer to bottle-feed, it is best not to make any final decision until the baby is born (see p.69). If you can, seek out a lactation consultant who breast-fed successfully herself and listen to her advice.

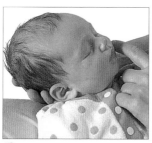

1 △ Your baby will instinctively search for the nipple to find food – the so-called rooting reflex. Encourage this by stroking the baby's cheek.

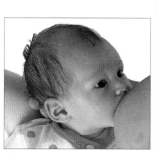

2 △ Once latched on, baby doesn't so much suck as "milk" with his jaws pressed on your milk supply at the base of the areola (area around nipple).

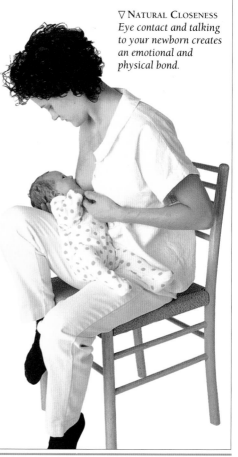

▽ NATURAL CLOSENESS
Eye contact and talking to your newborn creates an emotional and physical bond.

30 PRACTICAL MATERNITY WARDROBE

For the first six months of your pregnancy many of your regular clothes will be wearable, provided they are loose-fitting. However, there is nothing like buying a new wardrobe to boost morale – and you don't have to buy special maternity outfits. Bear in mind that you tend to get hotter more quickly during pregnancy, so choose lightweight cotton (or other natural fiber) items. Avoid tight-fitting clothes.

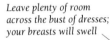

Leave plenty of room across the bust of dresses; your breasts will swell

◁ **LOOSE CLOTHES**
Oversized, baggy T-shirts, shirts, sweatshirts, and sweaters are comfortable. Choose the largest size.

Clothes must be loose around the waist

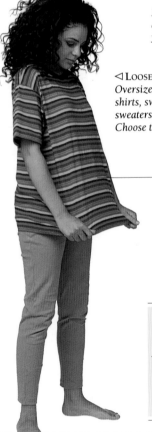

Choose sweatpants with adjustable waist cords that you can loosen as your waist expands

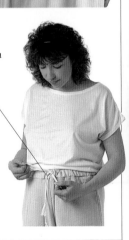

SHOE SUPPORT
Wear comfortable, low-heeled, but not flat, shoes. Avoid shoes with laces which will only become a nuisance later on in your pregnancy.

31 BUYING A NURSING BRA

You will need at least two nursing bras if you want to breast-feed after birth. Wait until after week 36; your breasts will swell at the end of pregnancy. There are two main types: front-opening bras that open to expose the nipple area only; and those that unfasten at the front to expose the whole breast. The latter allow the baby to feel as much of the breast as possible while sucking.

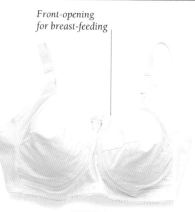

Front-opening for breast-feeding

NURSING BRA

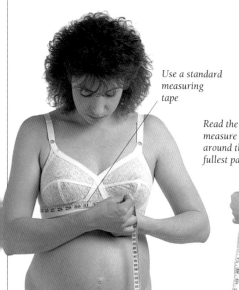

Use a standard measuring tape

1 △ At about week 36, put on a normal pregnancy bra and measure under your breasts with a standard measuring tape to find out your bra size.

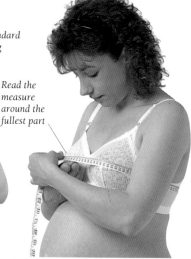

Read the measure around the fullest part

2 △ Measure around the fullest part of your breasts for the correct cup size. If in doubt, ask a salesperson in a maternity department to help you.

32 PACKING YOUR SUITCASE

A month before your due date, check that everything is ready for the baby. This is the best time to pack for the hospital, and think about what you will need if you plan to have your baby at home. Make sure you don't take too many things to the hospital; there may not be very much storage space in the maternity ward. It could be worth checking with the hospital first: some hospitals provide a list of what to take with you and even some of the items on it.

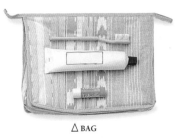

△ BAG

PERSONAL ITEMS
Make sure to include a toothbrush, toothpaste, lip balm, small sponge, deodorant, talcum powder, soap, washcloths, and towel.

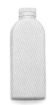

△ TALCUM POWDER

▽ SPONGE

△ DEODORANT

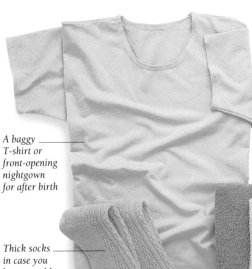

A baggy T-shirt or front-opening nightgown for after birth

Thick socks in case you become cold during labor

TOWEL, WASHCLOTHS & SOAP ▽

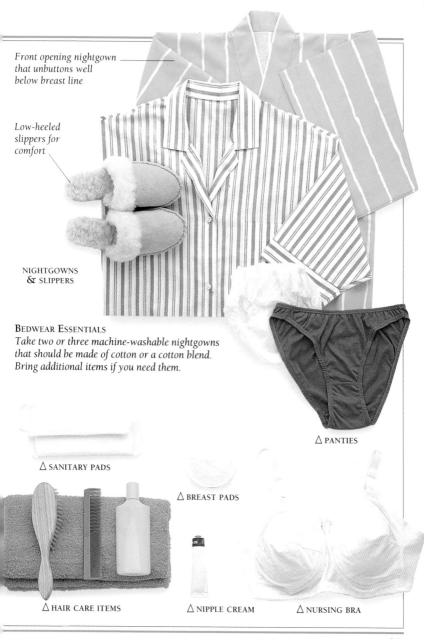

Front opening nightgown that unbuttons well below breast line

Low-heeled slippers for comfort

NIGHTGOWNS & SLIPPERS

BEDWEAR ESSENTIALS
Take two or three machine-washable nightgowns that should be made of cotton or a cotton blend. Bring additional items if you need them.

△ PANTIES

△ SANITARY PADS

△ BREAST PADS

△ HAIR CARE ITEMS

△ NIPPLE CREAM

△ NURSING BRA

33 RELATING TO YOUR FETUS

Both mother and father can benefit emotionally by trying to discover what the baby is experiencing before it is born. The fetus can feel, see, hear, and experience its mother's emotions through the release of chemicals such as endorphins (if you are happy). It kicks and punches in response, so talk to it, feel it, and soothe it with touches from the outside.

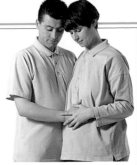

GENTLE TOUCHES & RUBS

34 FETUS KICK CHART

The number of kicks a fetus makes in a six-hour period can be an indication of its well-being during the third trimester. Make a chart like the one below to indicate the time by which five kicks are felt. If you are getting less than five movements within the time frame noted, this should be marked in the bottom panel.

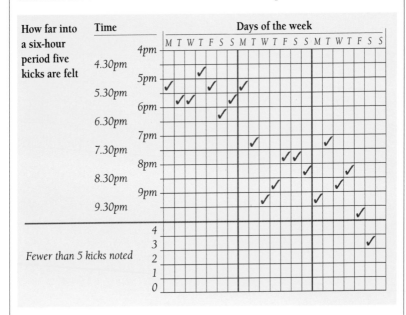

How far into a six-hour period five kicks are felt	Time	Days of the week																				
		M	T	W	T	F	S	S	M	T	W	T	F	S	S	M	T	W	T	F	S	S
	4pm																					
	4.30pm				✓																	
	5pm					✓																
	5.30pm	✓			✓																	
	6pm		✓	✓			✓															
	6.30pm						✓															
	7pm								✓								✓					
	7.30pm									✓	✓											
	8pm											✓						✓				
	8.30pm													✓					✓			
	9pm												✓		✓							
	9.30pm																				✓	
	4																					
	3																				✓	
Fewer than 5 kicks noted	2																					
	1																					
	0																					

35 GAINING STRENGTH

Make sure your diet has enough calcium (lowfat cheese, white bread, yogurt), protein (poultry, fish, peanut butter), vitamin C (orange, Brussels sprouts, tomatoes), fiber (wholegrain bread, beans, raisins), folic acid (broccoli, spinach), and iron (tuna fish, spinach, dried apricots). Try to eat some of the following each day: cheese, spinach, oranges, raisins, sardines, chicken, and fish.

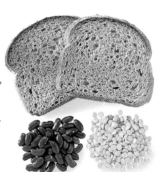

CALCIUM-RICH FOODS ▷
Foods such as sardines, farmer cheese, and yogurt help the healthy development of baby's bones and teeth. You will need twice as much calcium as normal.

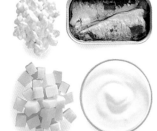

△ WHOLE GRAINS
So-called complex carbohydrates include cooked barley and brown rice, wholegrain or soy-flour bread, kidney beans, chickpeas, lentils, and peas. These provide fiber and help prevent constipation – a common complaint in pregnancy.

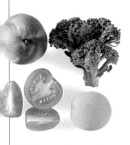

△ VITAMIN A-RICH FOODS
Green leafy and red or yellow vegetables, such as broccoli and tomato, help the baby's central nervous system develop.

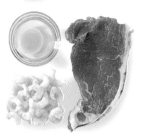

△ PROTEIN-RICH FOODS
Hard cheese, milk, yogurt, lamb, and fish are among the foods that provide first-class protein. Choose lean cuts of meat to avoid fat.

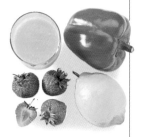

△ VITAMIN C-RICH FOODS
Items such as red peppers, strawberries, and oranges will help you build up a rich placenta and assist in fighting infections.

36 LOOKING AFTER YOUR BODY

MODERATE EXERCISE

You need to care for your body more during pregnancy than ever before, as it copes with the additional pressures and hormonal changes. Plenty of rest, a sensible diet, gentle exercise (especially swimming), and relaxation techniques all help keep your body fit and your mind relaxed.

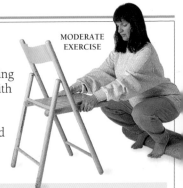

Symptoms & How to Treat Them

Complaint	What to do	Complaint	What to do
Breathlessness Growing baby puts pressure on diaphragm in later months; you feel breathless even when you talk	Rest as much as you can; try crouching if there's no chair to lean on; use an extra pillow at night. Consult doctor	**Sweating** Caused by increased blood flow to skin. Sweating after very little exertion; hot and sweaty at night	Wear cotton clothing and avoid man-made materials; drink plenty of fluids, especially water, and open windows at night
Feeling faint You feel dizzy and unstable and need to sit or lie down; this is because your blood pressure is lower in pregnancy	Don't stand still too long; sit down and put your head between your knees; get up slowly from a hot bath or from lying down	**Swollen and stiff fingers** Slight swellings in hot weather and stiff swollen fingers in mornings; rings may not fit	Rest often with your feet up; stretch feet gently and raise hands above head; flex each finger; see doctor if marked and persistent
Cramps Painful muscle contractions, usually in calves and feet, often at night. Leg stretch, with toes down, often starts it	Massage and rub the affected calf or foot; walk around to ease circulation. Bend foot up toward knee. Get plenty of calcium	**Varicose veins** Aching legs with the veins in the calves and thighs painful and swollen; likely in later pregnancy or if overweight	Rest with your feet raised on a cushion or two; tuck a pillow in the small of the back; support hose may help

37 LIFESTYLE CHANGES

Throughout your pregnancy, avoid any medication (unless otherwise directed by your doctor), give up smoking, and eliminate alcohol. Passive smoking is also a hazard, so stay out of smoky atmospheres. Avoid contact with raw meats and dog or cat feces.

MEDICINES

38 HAZARDS AT WORK

Certain jobs bring certain risks, such as X-ray machines at dentists, so you need to be conscious of your work environment: for instance, is it a factory with noxious chemicals such as dry-cleaning fluids, paint fumes, or solvents? Is the machinery excessively loud? Modern computer screens are not harmful. As at home, avoid exposure to cigarette smoke in the workplace.

39 PLANNING AHEAD AT WORK

As soon as you discover that you are pregnant:
▪ Check out your maternity leave rights and discuss maternity benefits with your employer.

▪ Give your insurance company a call to determine benefits.
▪ Ask your doctor for advice on how close to your due date it is advisable for you to work.

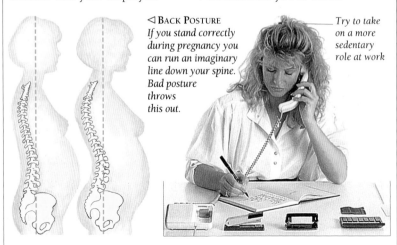

◁ BACK POSTURE
If you stand correctly during pregnancy you can run an imaginary line down your spine. Bad posture throws this out.

Try to take on a more sedentary role at work

OPTIONS FOR BIRTH

40 HOSPITAL BIRTH

Most births take place in a hospital, in special maternity units. This is because most doctors believe that the hospital is the safest place for a baby to be born. All the equipment and expertise is available for administering pain relief, for monitoring baby's progress, and for intervening in the birth if necessary.

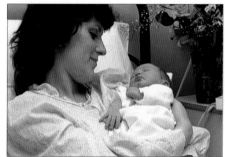

△ HOSPITAL REASSURANCE
You may find the support of hospital staff and other mothers reassuring. Emergency medical care is also on hand.

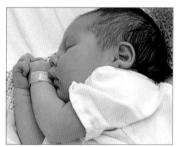

△ HOSPITAL STAYS
New laws in many states ensure that mothers may stay in hospital for 48 hours after a vaginal delivery.

41 HOSPITAL BIRTH OPTIONS

Well before your due date, tour the hospital (these tours are often part of Lamaze classes). Many hospitals now feature attractive birthing suites so that you can labor, deliver, and recover all in the same room. Some valuable features to look for: a private bathroom, a place for your partner to sleep so that he can stay with you during recovery, and 24-hour visiting.

42 HOME BIRTH CHECKLIST

If you decide on a home birth, the doctor or midwife who is going to deliver your baby will want to check beforehand that the room in which you plan to have the baby has all the necessary facilities. For a home delivery you will need:

- a well-lit, warm room;
- a bed accessible from both sides and in good light;
- plenty of hot water;
- a washable, low-dust floor – cover any carpet with protective sheeting;
- a plastic sheet to put over the mattress;
- plenty of pitchers and bowls to hold water if there is no sink in the room.

◁ THINGS YOU NEED
You will also need to have a bedpan, a bucket for soiled dressings, a soft towel to wrap baby in, two large basins, and a water pitcher. Plenty of hot water is also essential.

43 HOME BIRTH BENEFITS

If you are healthy, under 35, and have had a normal pregnancy, and one or two normal births without complications, then home birth is probably safe for you. It may even be safer because there is less risk of infection (the average home has fewer germs than most hospitals). You may feel more relaxed and calmer about breast-feeding. Your older children may also accept the newborn more readily.

44 HOME BIRTH PROBLEMS

It can be difficult to arrange a home birth, because most doctors are unwilling to deliver at home, especially if they feel there is any possiblity of problems arising needing hospital facilities. Also, with other children around it can be difficult to rest at home after the baby's birth. You are continually "on call" in your own home, however supportive your partner and family are.

45 WATER DURING LABOR

During labor, if your water has not broken, a warm bath can help you relax and often seems to ease the pain. Some hospitals provide labor pools that are large enough for you to move around in and find a comfortable position with the water supporting your body. Some people believe that giving birth in water makes it a gentler and less traumatic experience for the baby. However, others consider water birth a poor idea – it is potentially too dangerous because the baby will be unable to breathe if kept underwater and may even drown.

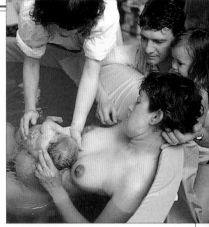

△ LABOR POOL
A warm bath or shower can help ease the pain of labor. If your hospital provides these facilities, then consider taking advantage of them.

46 CONSIDER YOUR OPTIONS

Whether you choose to give birth at the hospital or at home, your labor will be an exciting but challenging event. Be sure to choose a doctor or midwife who you feel confident will guide you sensibly, sympathetically, and expertly through your labor. Discuss with your partner, doctor, or midwife the options for the birthing situation that appeal to you, and are most appropriate to your medical circumstances, to ensure you are choosing the calmest, most comfortable, and safest environment.

47 NATURAL CHILDBIRTH

Based on the principle that pain is linked to fear and tension, natural childbirth relies on relaxation and breathing techniques. These techniques must be practiced at prenatal classes and at home. What natural childbirth cannot do is guarantee pain-free birth.

BE REALISTIC ▷
It's fine to hope for a childbirth without pain relief or medical intervention, but be prepared to accept pain-killers if needed.

FIRST STAGES OF LABOR

48 KNOWING YOU ARE IN LABOR

You will probably recognize labor when it starts, but you may confuse the first contractions of labor with those that may occur in the last weeks of pregnancy. Look for these signs:

- A show, which is a plug of thick, blood-stained mucus that blocks the neck of the womb and passes out of the vagina.

- The bag of amniotic fluid that surrounds the baby, your "water," breaks. It may be sudden, but is more often a trickle; as the baby's head moves, fluid leaks.

- Contractions may start as back pain, or you may feel chilled, nauseous, or have diarrhea. If you are unsure whether you are in labor, don't hesitate to call your doctor.

FINDING SOME COMFORT ▷
Assume the most comfortable position for you to relieve the pain of contractions and then to relax.

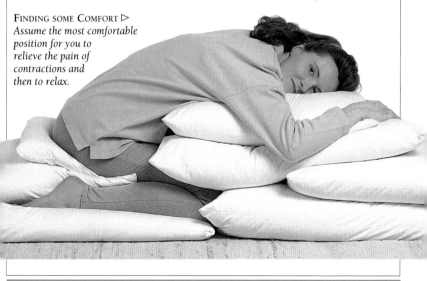

49 FALSE STARTS

Your uterus contracts during the pregnancy; contractions become stronger and more noticeable in the last few weeks (these are known as Braxton-Hicks contractions, and are easily mistaken for the first signs of labor). But when true contractions start they occur at fairly regular intervals, gradually growing stronger and more frequent. Timing your contractions will help you determine whether it is the real thing.

50 TIMING YOUR CONTRACTIONS

Contractions can start off as a dull backache, or you may experience shooting pains down your thighs. They will eventually feel like severe menstrual cramps. When the contractions seem to be regular, time them over the space of an hour, noting when each one starts and when it ends. They will gradually become stronger and more frequent (*see below*).

51 ARRIVING AT THE HOSPITAL

True contractions will last for at least 40 seconds as labor sets in. At first you may get four contractions an hour with intervals of between 15 to 20 minutes. Once the contractions come very frequently, say every five minutes, or are painful, go to the hospital. (Call your doctor first if you have time.) You may feel panic-stricken, but stay as calm as you can and try to work with your body. Once you reach the hospital you will see a nurse who will ask some questions. Having your partner with you will help.

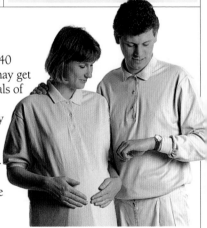

MONITOR YOUR CONTRACTIONS

52 FIRST CHECKS & QUESTIONS

On arrival at hospital the nurse or doctor will ask you about the frequency of contractions. She also will ask if you have had a show (the plug of thick blood-stained mucus that blocks the neck of the womb and passes out of the vagina as labor starts); or if your water (that surrounds the baby) has broken.

53 THE CERVIX IN LABOR

The cervix is kept closed by a ring of muscles. Other muscles run from the cervix up and over the uterus. These muscles contract during labor, drawing the cervix into the uterus and then stretching it so that it dilates (opens up) wide enough for the baby's head to pass through. The more the cervix dilates, the closer you are to delivery.

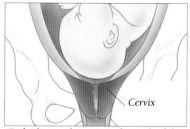

1 △ The tough cervix is the neck of the uterus. It is a thick-walled canal about 2.5 cm long. During labor it starts to open up to about 10 cm.

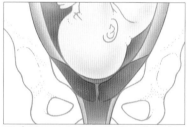

2 △ The cervix is gradually softened by hormone changes, and the contractions also slowly soften, pull up, and efface (thin) the cervix.

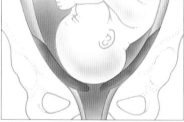

3 △ During the first stages of labor the cervix eventually becomes fully effaced. After this stage, stronger contractions dilate it.

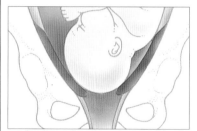

4 △ When it has dilated to a width of 7 cm the doctor or nurse can feel the cervix stretched out to form a thin lip around the baby's head.

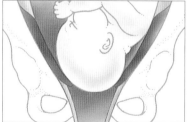

5 △ At 10 cm, when the doctor or nurse cannot feel the cervix, it is fully dilated. The vagina and uterus have become one continuous "birth canal."

54 GETTING COMFORTABLE

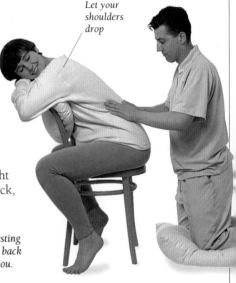

Let your shoulders drop

Different positions are comfortable at different stages, so try out a few for the first stage. You could practice them beforehand so that you can follow your body's natural cues more easily. A partner or other birth assistant can be a physical as well as emotional support, supporting your weight when needed, rubbing your back, and soothing and holding you.

SIT DOWN
Lean forward with legs wide apart, resting your head on your folded arms on the back of the chair while your partner rubs you.

55 STAYING UPRIGHT

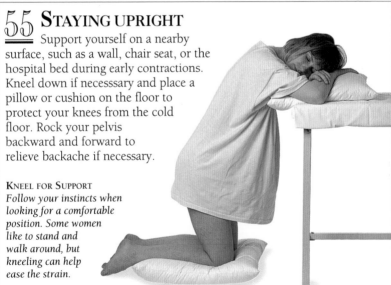

Support yourself on a nearby surface, such as a wall, chair seat, or the hospital bed during early contractions. Kneel down if necesssary and place a pillow or cushion on the floor to protect your knees from the cold floor. Rock your pelvis backward and forward to relieve backache if necessary.

KNEEL FOR SUPPORT
Follow your instincts when looking for a comfortable position. Some women like to stand and walk around, but kneeling can help ease the strain.

56 SITTING FORWARD

You may find it most comfortable to sit down facing the back of a chair with your legs straddled on either side. If you choose to assume this position, lean over the back using a cushion or pillow to prop up your head and arms. Rest your head on your folded arms. Keep your knees apart. You can also put a cushion on the seat of the chair. Alternatively, to keep your body suppported, you could lean against your partner, a door, or a counter or sink.

BACK SUPPORT
When sitting, always make sure your back is straight, but don't hesitate to sit on cushions or pillows, or lean against your birth attendant to keep your back supported.

57 KNEELING FORWARD

You can ease your discomfort by kneeling down on the floor with your legs apart, balancing forward on a pile of cushions or pillows. Try to stay as upright as possible and sit to one side between contractions. Raising your bottom with your head still on the floor (on pillows) may help relieve backache (caused by the baby's head pressing against your abdomen). Do not arch your back.

EASE PRESSURE
This kneeling position can help take the pressure off your lower back.

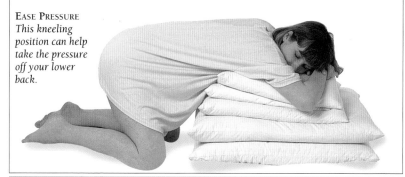

58 BACKACHE RELIEF

Kneeling on all fours on the floor with your back straight, not arched, can help you work through contractions and backache. You may find a mattress more comfortable or, if that is not practical, place some pillows or cushions under your knees. Between contractions lean forward on folded arms or sit back on your heels.

TILT FORWARD
Tilt your pelvis to and fro and, between contractions, relax forward and rest your head in your arms. Leaning forward like this helps take the baby's weight off your back.

Rock your pelvis back and forth

Keep your back straight

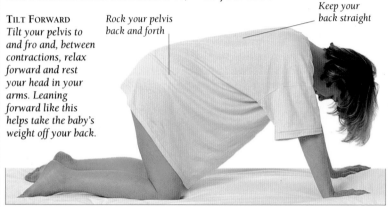

59 LOWER BACK MASSAGE

Your partner should massage the base of your spine using the heel of his hand to make firm, circular movements. A sprinkle of talcum powder can prevent friction rub of skin on skin. Lower back massage will help calm and reassure you as well as relieve backache.

PARTNER'S HELPING HANDS
Your partner's hands will soothe you and take your mind off the pain.

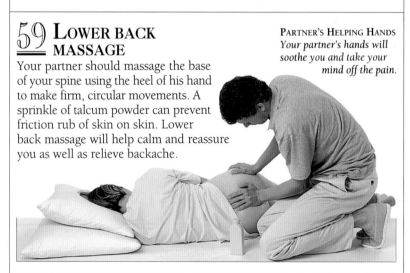

60 WHAT YOUR PARTNER CAN DO

A birth partner's main role is to offer emotional and physical comfort and support to the mother, and to give praise and encouragement. It is important, too, to stay calm if she gets annoyed and distressed. Remind her of her breathing exercises, mop her brow, hold her hand, hug her around the shoulders, massage her back, and give her sips of water or ice chips.

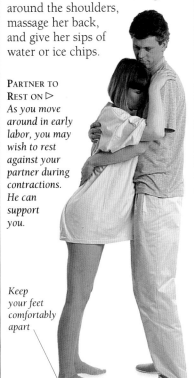

PARTNER TO REST ON ▷
As you move around in early labor, you may wish to rest against your partner during contractions. He can support you.

Keep your feet comfortably apart

61 BREATHING FOR THE FIRST STAGE

Breathe deeply and evenly at the start and end of each contraction – in through the nose, out through the mouth. When the contraction peaks, take lighter and shallower breaths, breathing through your mouth throughout.

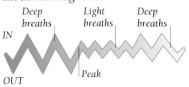

Deep breaths   *Light breaths*   *Deep breaths*

IN

OUT   *Peak*

SHALLOW BREATHING
Breathe through your mouth at the peak – but not for too long or you will feel dizzy.

62 BREATHING FOR THE SECOND STAGE

Contractions may last a minute now and come every minute: to work through these say "huff, huff, blow," taking in short in and out breaths. Then blow out a longer breath. When the pain has passed, release a slow, even breath.

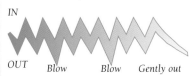

IN

OUT   *Blow*   *Blow*   *Gently out*

BREATHING CONTROL
Short intakes and outtakes of breath can help during the second stage of labor; it also eases the urge to push.

63 SELF-HELP CHECKLIST

As the contractions become stronger and more frequent, try a variety of the positions you have already rehearsed (see pp.40–43). Some will work better than others.

If you want to lie down, do so on your side, not on your back, and have plenty of pillows supporting your head and thighs. Remember your breathing exercises.

Dealing with contractions

- Keep moving between contractions to help you cope physically with the pain.
- Concentrate on your breathing to take your mind off the contractions.
- Relax between contractions to save your energy.
- Urinate often so your bladder does not get in the way of the baby.

- Try to stay upright so the baby's head sits firmly on the cervix. This makes your contractions stronger.
- Sing, or let out a moan or cry to release the pain. Don't hold back or feel embarrassed.
- Concentrate on a fixed spot, site, or object as a way of distracting your mind from the pain.

64 WHEN TO PUSH & WHEN NOT TO PUSH

The hardest time during labor can be at the end of the first stage, known as "transition," when contractions are strongest but before the cervix has fully dilated. In this stage you want to push, but it may be too early and the cervix can get bruised and swollen. Tell the doctor or nurse that you feel ready and they will check internally to make sure.

STOP YOURSELF FROM PUSHING
If the doctor says you are not fully dilated, say "huff, huff, blow" in this position in time with your breathing.

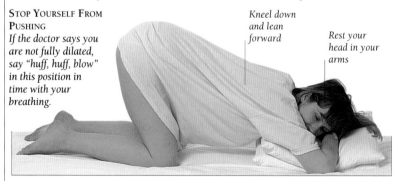

Kneel down and lean forward

Rest your head in your arms

PAIN RELIEF

65 OPTIONS FOR PAIN RELIEF

However determined you may have been not to take pain relief before labor, once you start to feel the contractions, the discomfort may be more than you anticipated. Just remember the options are there to help you. Some drugs enter the baby's bloodstream, others don't. They are safe for you and your baby, and will ease the pain should you require one or all of them.

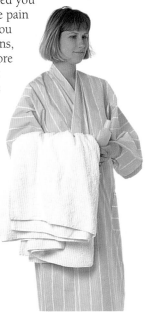

CLEAR CHOICES
State your preferences for pain relief very clearly. It is a good idea to discuss options with your doctor beforehand.

66 DEMEROL

This is a pain-relieving drug that will make you calm, relaxed, and somewhat sleepy, but still aware of what is going on. You may feel sick or "drunk" and have no desire to move around. The drug is normally injected in the buttocks and takes 20 minutes to have an effect. Demerol (or meperidine) lasts for a few hours and is often given in the first stage of labor. It can cause sleepiness in your baby as well, but this will wear off soon after the delivery.

67 EPIDURAL ANESTHESIA

An epidural completely numbs the nerves of the lower body for about two hours by means of an anesthetic injected into the spine. It is highly effective for relieving pain but must be timed very carefully so that the effects have worn off by the second stage of labor, or you will take longer to push out.

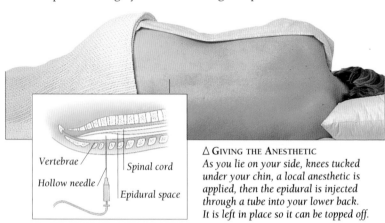

Vertebrae
Hollow needle
Spinal cord
Epidural space

△ GIVING THE ANESTHETIC
As you lie on your side, knees tucked under your chin, a local anesthetic is applied, then the epidural is injected through a tube into your lower back. It is left in place so it can be topped off.

68 INHALATION

Better known as "gas and air," inhalation analgesics are a mixture of oxygen and gas, which gives pain relief and is less intrusive than an epidural. It is also self-ministered. You take deep breaths through a hand-held mask as you feel a contraction coming on. The edge of the pain is reduced and you may feel light-headed.

BREATHING IN ▷
Your partner can give you support as you regulate the amount of gas that you inhale. You can also move around freely.

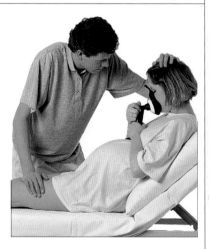

69 TENS

This electronic sensor heightens the body's natural defenses of pain relief by sending impulses of electric currents to your back. Pads containing electrodes are stuck to your back over the nerves that supply the womb. These pads are linked to a control panel you hold to intensify or lessen the current strength. It is useful for mild labor pains.

SELF CONTROL
You control the switch and you can move around with TENS. It is not harmful and it is easy to use.

70 MONITORING YOUR LABOR

During labor the midwife or nurse will place either a hand-held fetal stethoscope, sonicaid, or electronic fetal monitoring (EFM) instrument on your stomach to record the baby's heartbeat. EFM is not painful but it does restrict you to the bed as monitoring pads are attached to your abdomen to measure contractions.

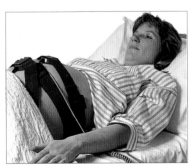

STRAPPED & PADDED
As you lie on pillows, heartbeat and contractions are measured on a paper print-out attached to the monitor.

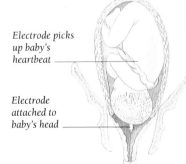

Electrode picks up baby's heartbeat

Electrode attached to baby's head

PICKING UP THE HEARTBEAT
An electrode is attached to the presenting part of the baby (usually the head). It may cause a minor bruise or rash.

SECOND STAGE OF LABOR

71 SITTING UPRIGHT FOR DELIVERY

Once the cervix has dilated and you can push, the second stage of labor has begun. This is when you can add your own impetus to the contractions and help push the baby out. The contractions may be stronger. Sitting upright or lying back with legs up are common delivery positions. Pushing is hard work, but your nurse or midwife and partner can help you to adopt the most comfortable position for you. They will encourage you to push when necessary.

SITTING COMFORTABLY
Sit on the bed propped up by pillows, a bean bag, a wedge, or even your partner. Keep your chin down, and grip under your thighs as you push. Lean forward and keep your legs apart. Relax back into the pillows between contractions.

UPRIGHT
Try to be as upright as you can when pushing, so you are working with gravity, rather than against it.

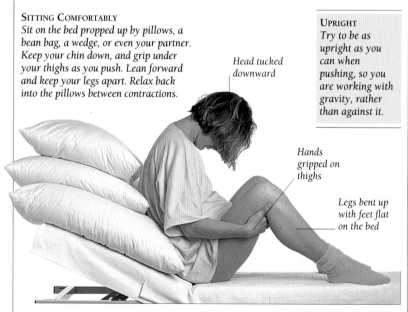

Head tucked downward

Hands gripped on thighs

Legs bent up with feet flat on the bed

72 SQUATTING FOR DELIVERY

An excellent position for delivery, squatting opens the pelvis wide and uses gravity to help you push out the baby. You may find it tiring, however, after a while. Any back support from your partner can be invaluable here and also help you to relax.

PARTNER SUPPORT
If your partner sits on the edge of a chair, with his legs apart, you can squat between his knees and rest your arms on his thighs for support and between contractions.

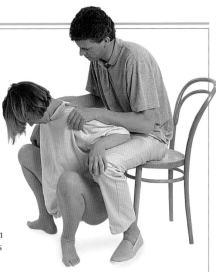

73 KNEELING FOR DELIVERY

Kneeling may be less tiring than squatting, and it is also a good position to push from. You may find that alternating this position with kneeling down on all fours gives you some extra relief. Whether kneeling or squatting, try to keep you back straight at all times. Your partner and midwife or nurse will guide and support you.

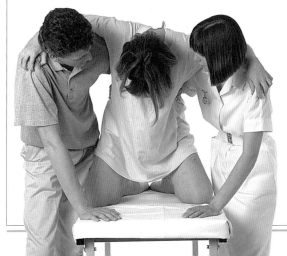

PARTNER ROLE
Your partner should give you physical support and emotional encouragement and tell you what's going on all the time.

◁ **HELPING HANDS**
Your partner and nurse can help you feel more stable by supporting you under your arms on either side while you squat.

74 BREATHING & PUSHING

When you want to push, take a deep breath and hold it for a short time as you bear down. Between pushes, take a few deep calm breaths.

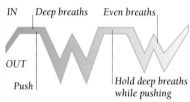

IN | Deep breaths | Even breaths
OUT
Push | Hold deep breaths while pushing

△ **BREATHING FOR THE SECOND STAGE**
You may want to push several times during a contraction. Do what your body tells you and relax slowly after the contraction.

75 NO URGE TO PUSH

Many books on childbirth tell the woman that at some point during her labor she will feel an irresistible urge to push. The truth is that although this is nearly always true, some women never have this feeling. This means that at each contraction they have to make a conscious effort to push – their bodies do not tell them to do so. The same thing happens if the effects of an epidural have not worn off by the second stage. Even if you feel no urge, you can still push effectively. The doctor or midwife will tell you when to push.

76 BEING OVERDUE: WHAT HAPPENS

If more than two weeks have passed since the baby's due date or it shows signs of being distressed; if the placenta starts to fail; or if you have high blood pressure, putting the baby at risk, labor may be induced, that is, started artificially. This is done by inserting a suppository into the vagina, rupturing the membranes, or giving a hormone, via an IV, which makes the uterus contract. You will be consulted about this beforehand.

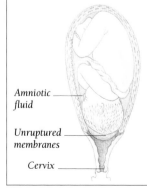

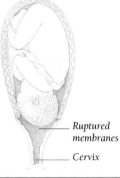

◁ **INTACT MEMBRANES**
The membranes usually rupture naturally, releasing the amniotic fluid that has cushioned the baby during pregnancy.

RUPTURED MEMBRANES ▷
With a surgical tool a small opening is made. This ruptures the membrane so that the baby's head moves against the cervix.

Amniotic fluid

Unruptured membranes

Cervix

Ruptured membranes

Cervix

THE BIRTH

77 THE BIRTH FROM START TO DELIVERY

The climax of labor has arrived: soon you will be able to touch the baby's head for the first time as it emerges. You will not damage yourself or the baby as you push during contractions because vaginal walls are elastic and made of folds so they can stretch to allow the baby through. After delivery you will probably feel a sense of intense relief, tinged with great emotion and joy and a feeling of overwhelming tenderness toward your newborn baby.

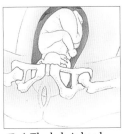

1 △ The baby's head moves to the vaginal opening. The head can be seen during contractions.

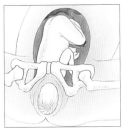

2 △ The head "crowns" (the top is now visible). You stop pushing and "relax" with panting breaths.

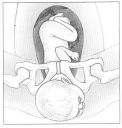

3 △ The head is born face down; the doctor checks the umbilical cord, then the baby turns her head to one side.

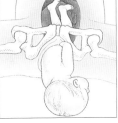

4 △ The doctor cleans her face, and the body slides out within two contractions. The doctor gives you the baby.

78 AFTER THE BIRTH

The placenta is delivered and checked by the doctor. You will be cleaned up (and stitched if necessary); the baby's Apgar score will be recorded (see p.53) and the umbilical cord (still attached) will now be clamped and cut. You can then hold her for a few minutes.

79 YOUR NEW BABY

Do not be dismayed if your baby doesn't look perfect – few babies do at birth. He will seem smaller than you imagined and very vulnerable. His head shape may seem strange and he may be covered with a white greasy substance called vernix. Most of these peculiarities will disappear after baby is about two weeks old. The main features to be prepared for are:

- The strange shape of the head caused by the pressure of the birth on the fontanel (top of the head).
- The eyes will be blue, and true eye color may not develop until baby is six months old.
- Squinting is common, so don't worry if he appears cross-eyed.
- The hands and feet may seem bluish because circulation is not working fully. They will turn pink.
- A baby's breasts may be swollen and even leak a little milk. This is normal in both sexes. The swelling goes down in a few days.

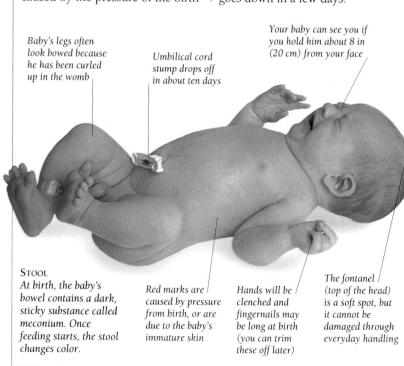

Baby's legs often look bowed because he has been curled up in the womb

Umbilical cord stump drops off in about ten days

Your baby can see you if you hold him about 8 in (20 cm) from your face

STOOL
At birth, the baby's bowel contains a dark, sticky substance called meconium. Once feeding starts, the stool changes color.

Red marks are caused by pressure from birth, or are due to the baby's immature skin

Hands will be clenched and fingernails may be long at birth (you can trim these off later)

The fontanel (top of the head) is a soft spot, but it cannot be damaged through everyday handling

80 NEWBORN SKIN FEATURES

Seeing your baby's skin for the first time – with its spots, red marks, blotches, other blemishes, and changes of color – may cause you concern, especially as a first-time mother, but it shouldn't. Skin marks are normal because the systems of his body are not yet working properly. If anything does concern you, ask your doctor or pediatrician.

■ Rashes are very common and most will vanish of their own accord in time.

■ Peeling skin on hands and feet will disappear after a couple of days.

■ Most birthmarks will vanish, including "storkmarks" around the eyes and head, which go away after a year; strawberry marks, which are larger, usually disappear after five years.

■ Any traces of downy body hair will disappear.

■ Greasy white vernix is the substance that protects the baby's skin in the uterus; it may cover him completely. It can be wiped off easily.

■ Your baby may have a good head of hair or may be bald; either is perfectly normal.

81 WHAT IS THE APGAR TEST?

Within a minute of the birth, your baby is given five quick tests to assess his health. This is called the Apgar Test (named after the doctor who originally devised it).

■ Overall pink color shows the lungs are working properly.

■ Pulse indicates a strong and regular heartbeat.

■ Facial expressions reveal alert responses to stimuli.

■ Limb activity confirms muscle tone.

■ Respiration shows health of lungs. The test is repeated after 5 minutes.

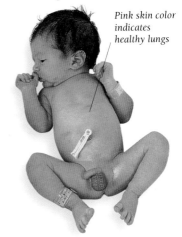

Pink skin color indicates healthy lungs

HOW THE SCORE WORKS
Most babies score between 7 and 10 (2 points for each test). Over 7 means your baby is in "good condition." Under 4 means he may need resuscitation, but a retest usually shows improvements.

82 FIRST CHECKS FOR YOUR BABY

Your baby is given a more specific examination by the doctor or nurse (after the quick Apgar Test, *see p. 53*). His facial features and body condition are checked over, as is his back and anus, fingers and toes, and the umbilical cord. Then the baby's head is measured, with checks made on the fontanel (soft spot) and the roof of his mouth. Below are the main areas examined:

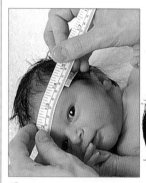

1 △ The doctor or nurse measures the head, checks the fontanel, and feels the roof of the mouth.

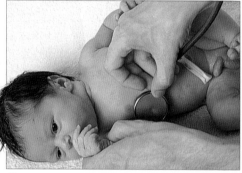

2 △ A stethoscope is used to listen to the heart and lungs to see if they are working normally. Heart murmurs are common among newborn babies and do not usually indicate any defect.

3 ▽ Hands are placed on the tummy to check the abdominal organs are the right size. The pulse is felt in the baby's groin.

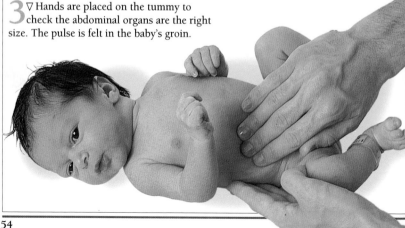

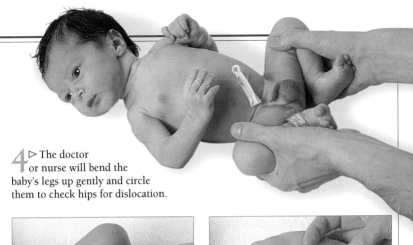

4 ▷ The doctor or nurse will bend the baby's legs up gently and circle them to check hips for dislocation.

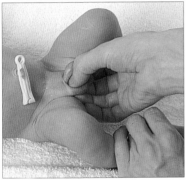

5 △ The genitals are checked for any abnormalities. If you have a boy the doctor will be looking to see if both testicles have descended. They are often pulled up into the groin. The genitals on newborns look large on both male and female babies.

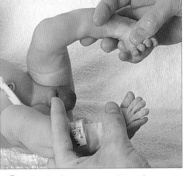

6 △ The limbs are moved gently to and fro, and the lower legs and feet checked to make sure that they are in alignment and that the legs are the right length (and that the baby does not suffer from foot problems).

7 ▷ A thumb is run down the baby's back to make sure that all the vertebrae are in place along the spine.

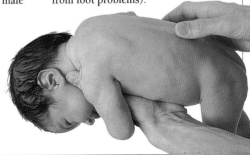

83 NEWBORN BEHAVIOR

At first your baby will spend a lot of time curled up (just as in the womb) with fists tightly closed. When she lies on her back, her head will loll from side to side because a newborn baby's head is too heavy for her back and neck muscles to support. By the time she is one week old she will be able to raise her head in small jerks when supported on your shoulder. At six weeks she may lift her head for a moment when on her tummy. If her hand happens to come into contact with her mouth, she will suck it which comforts her.

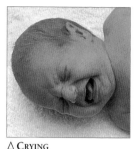

△ CRYING
This is her signal to tell you that she needs love, comfort, and probably feeding. Sudden movement, a loud noise, or turning on a bright light can trigger your baby's tears.

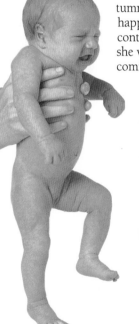

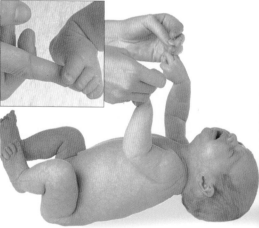

STEP REFLEX △
Once she can lift her head up, hold her under the arms and let her feet touch a firm surface; she will make stepping movements. Her toes will curl if touched.

GRASPING TIGHT △
This is a key reflex action to watch for. As you place your finger across her palm she will grasp it so tightly that her whole body weight can be supported.

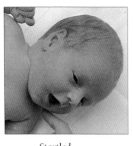

◁ **MOUTH REFLEXES**
Reflex movements are baby's way of protecting herself. The sucking reflex is very strong and is more like a chomping than a sucking. The rooting reflex can be triggered by stroking the cheek.

SOUNDING OFF
Light breathing noises, sneezes, and hiccups are common sounds for a baby. They do not mean that she has a cold. If you are still worried, have your doctor listen.

Startled limbs thrown straight out

MORO REFLEX △
If startled, a baby will suddenly spread her arms out like this as if to catch something. It is called the Moro reflex.

Hours of sleep and number of feeds per day for newborns

4 lb (2 kg) baby: awake for 7–8 feedings

7 lb (3 kg) baby: awake for 5–6 feedings

10 lb (4.5 kg) baby: awake for 4–5 feedings

| 0 | 5 | 10 | 15 | 20 |

Hours of sleep per day

◁ **SLEEP PATTERNS**
A newborn's sleeping habit depends on her weight and feeding needs. The less she weighs, the more she eats, which means less sleeping, and vice versa.

SPECIAL CARE & PROCEDURES

84 EPISIOTOMY

This is a small, surgical cut employed to widen the vaginal opening and prevent tears. Tears have ragged edges and heal less efficiently. An episiotomy may be used if the skin around your vaginal opening has not stretched enough, or if the baby is distressed or premature, or has a big head. A local anesthetic is given to numb your pelvic floor area and the cut is made at the peak of a contraction. This can cause discomfort and soreness later.

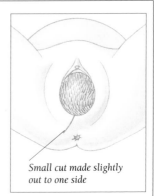

Small cut made slightly out to one side

85 ASSISTED DELIVERY

If your baby has a big head, or you cannot push the baby out, or he is in distress or breech, then forceps or suction may be used to assist delivery. You may be given both a local injection and episiotomy first, then the forceps are placed on either side of the baby's head, protecting it as it is gently pulled. You help by pushing.

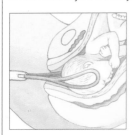

◁ **FORCEPS**
Old-fashioned but effective pulling implement that can leave temporary bruises on the baby's head.

VACUUM OR SUCTION ▷
A small metal cap, attached to a vacuum pump, is placed on the baby's head.

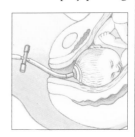

86 CESAREAN SECTION

The baby is delivered via the abdomen in a cesarean birth. You may know in advance that you are going to have one, or it may be an emergency operation. If planned, you can have a cesarean under an epidural anesthetic, so you can hold your baby right away; sometimes in emergencies, a general anesthetic may be required. The surgeon cuts across, drains away the amniotic fluid, and lifts out the baby, sometimes with forceps.

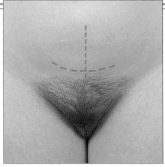

WHERE THE CUT IS MADE
An incision is made across the shaved pubic hair area. It takes 5 minutes from cut to birth; 20 minutes to stitch.

87 BREECH BIRTH

A breech baby is born bottom first and the largest part (the head) is born last. This means labor can be longer and more difficult. The baby's head size is measured by ultrasound. Breech birth must take place in a hospital since you will need an episiotomy, and forceps are often required. About 4 in 100 babies are breech.

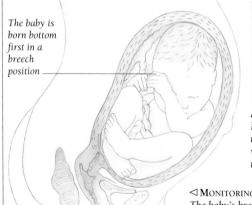

The baby is born bottom first in a breech position

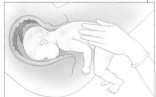

△ **DELIVERY OF THE LEGS**
First the baby's buttocks, and then his legs, are delivered. You will have an episiotomy before the delivery of the head.

◁ **MONITORING THE BREECH**
The baby's breech position and size of its head are monitored by ultrasound to check if it is small enough to fit through your pelvis.

88 TWINS

The sonogram at week 16 will reveal if you are having twins. Pregnancy and labor will progress normally, but twins will put extra strain on your body, and there is a greater likelihood of the babies lying abnormally in the womb and one of them being a breech. You will need to give birth in a hospital, since forceps and an epidural may be necessary. You will also have two second stages in labor: First you push one baby out, and then the other, about 10 to 30 minutes later.

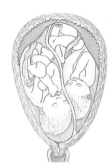

◁ IDENTICAL TWINS
A third of all twins are identical. They are always the same sex and usually share the placenta depending on how late the egg splits.

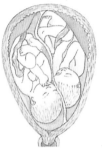

FRATERNAL TWINS ▷
These types of twins develop from separate fertilized eggs, and may or may not be of the same sex. Each has its own placenta.

89 BONDING

Babies needing special care need to bond with their mother (and father) just as strongly as any other. Many hospitals have rooms you can stay in to be near your baby so you can take part in her daily care. Special-care babies may look so small and vulnerable that you worry about touching them; but don't. All babies respond to loving handling.

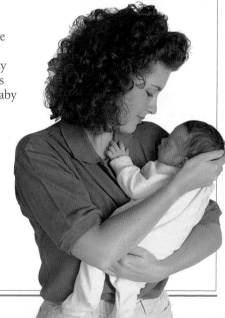

BUILDING A LOVING RELATIONSHIP
Bring her up close and talk and coo to her. Use eye contact and lots of cuddles and kisses to reassure and comfort her.

90 PREMATURE BABIES

Babies born before 37 weeks are described as premature and require special care at birth. They are more likely to have difficulties with breathing, feeding, and keeping warm, and will need to spend some time in an incubator. If your baby can suck, you will be able to to feed her normally. Otherwise, she will be fed through a tube that is passed through her nose or mouth and down straight into her stomach.

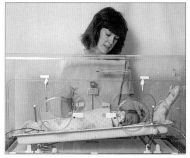

INCUBATOR
Incubators look unwelcoming, but they have portholes so you can touch your baby. The tilting tray helps breathing.

91 NEWBORN JAUNDICE

Many newborn babies suffer a mild condition that appears after three days in which their skin and the whites of their eyes turn slightly yellow. It is called jaundice and happens because a pigment called bilirubin develops faster than the liver can dispose of it. It usually clears up after a few days but exposure to sunlight through a window can help. Sometimes phototherapy (the use of special lights) is used to treat severe cases.

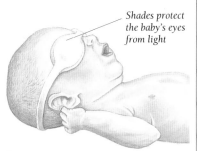

Shades protect the baby's eyes from light

PHOTOTHERAPY
If bilirubin levels are very high, the baby may be exposed to controlled amounts of ultraviolet light that break down the pigment levels in the skin.

92 SMALL-FOR-DATES BABIES

If a baby doesn't grow properly in the uterus and is small at birth, this is known as "small-for-dates." Smoking or poor diet can contribute, as can conditions such as diabetes that prevent the placenta from working properly. Such a baby will be carefully monitored and delivered early by induction or cesarean section.

GETTING BACK TO NORMAL

93 HOW TO COPE WITH THE BLUES

A few days after delivery, usually when the milk comes in, many women suffer postpartum depression. The sudden change in hormone levels is one cause for feeling low, as is the sense of anticlimax that often occurs after birth. These so-called "baby blues" and feelings of dejection and fatigue usually vanish after a few days. But if you feel very depressed or the depression lasts over a month, talk to your doctor. Very rarely, postpartum depression proves so severe that psychiatric care is necessary.

How you will feel

Problems	What to do
Afterpains Cramping pains in your stomach as the uterus contracts back to normal size	Take a mild pain medication such as acetominophen if the contractions are severe. The pain may last for several days
Bladder You will pass more water in the first days as your body loses the extra fluid gained in pregnancy	Try to urinate soon after birth even if it is difficult. Move around to encourage the flow. Soak in a warm bath. If you have stitches, pour warm water over them first
Bleeding From two to six weeks you will probably have vaginal bleeding. It is heavy and bright red at first, later brownish	Discharge may continue until the first period. Wear sanitary pads; do not use tampons since they can cause infection. Call your doctor if the discharge becomes heavier or bright red
Bowels For a day or more after the birth you may not want to empty your bowels. However, after this you will need to get your bowels working	Be active as soon as you can; walking around will start your bowels working. Drink plenty of water and eat high-fiber foods to stimulate your bowels. Holding a clean sanitary napkin against stitches may help

94 BODY RECOVERY & CHECKUP

It will take at least four weeks for your body to recover fully from the birth. By that time you will also be ready for your first important checkup, and baby's, with the doctor (see p.66):

- Your womb should have shrunk back to prepregnancy size.
- You may have started your periods again. The first one after the birth is often longer and heavier than usual.
- You should have begun some gentle exercises, particularly to strengthen the pelvic floor muscles.
- Your blood pressure, weight, and a sample of urine will be checked.

- Your breasts and stomach will be examined. The doctor will check that any stitches have healed.
- You may have an internal examination to ensure the size and position of the womb are normal, and you may be given a Pap test at this stage.
- The doctor will advise on appropriate forms of contraception, such as a diaphragm, an IUD, or condoms.
- You can also consult your doctor about other concerns, such as breast-feeding, diet, and fatigue.

95 BREAST & NIPPLE CARE

Take good care of your breasts – especially if you are breast-feeding. A good nursing bra with disposable breast pads is essential. Gently massage your breasts and expose them to the air; sore nipples heal more quickly this way. Wash your breasts with water and baby oil, but do not use soap, since it dries the skin. Pat them dry rather than rubbing. If the nipples are cracked or sore, apply baby lotion to a breast pad or use a calendula-based cream.

KEEP ON FEEDING ▷
If you encounter problems, such as leaking or engorged breasts, blocked ducts, or sore nipples, do not stop feeding, or you will make the problem worse. See your doctor.

96 TESTING YOUR PELVIC FLOOR

The pelvic floor is a hammock of muscles that supports the organs within the pelvis, a bony area that cradles and protects the baby in the womb. These muscles are stretched and weakened during pregnancy, often causing some leakage of urine. Three months after childbirth, if pelvic floor exercises are practiced regularly (*see right*), the muscles should be strong again. If urine still leaks, exercise for another month. See your doctor after that.

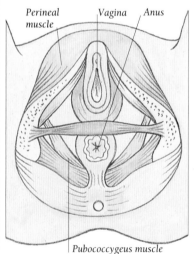

Perineal muscle   Vagina   Anus

Pubococcygeus muscle

PELVIC FLOOR MUSCLES
These support the bowel, bladder, and uterus, and they become stretched during pregnancy due to the weight of the fetus.

97 BODY RECOVERY EXERCISES

Start gentle exercises, especially those that will strengthen your pelvic floor, as soon as you can after delivery. With exercise, your figure can return to something like its prepregnancy shape in as little as three months. Your stomach muscles will not be as firm as before, though. If you have had a cesarean you will have to wait longer to start exercising. Always check with your doctor first.

SHAPING THE WAIST
Bending slowly to the left, raise your right arm over your head and pull your left arm down your left leg as far as you can. Hold. Relax. Repeat.

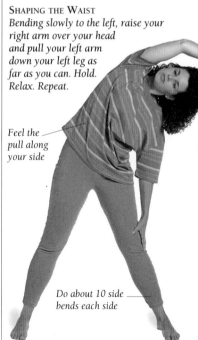

Feel the pull along your side

Do about 10 side bends each side

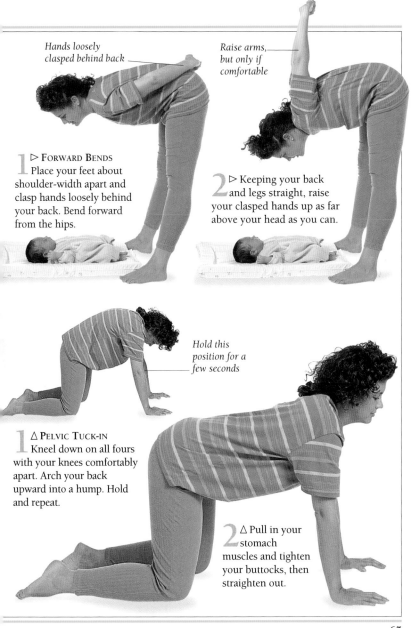

Hands loosely clasped behind back

Raise arms, but only if comfortable

1 ▷ FORWARD BENDS
Place your feet about shoulder-width apart and clasp hands loosely behind your back. Bend forward from the hips.

2 ▷ Keeping your back and legs straight, raise your clasped hands up as far above your head as you can.

Hold this position for a few seconds

1 △ PELVIC TUCK-IN
Kneel down on all fours with your knees comfortably apart. Arch your back upward into a hump. Hold and repeat.

2 △ Pull in your stomach muscles and tighten your buttocks, then straighten out.

98 YOUR BABY'S FIRST CHECKUP

At six weeks your baby will have her first major developmental checkup. Your doctor will begin with a general assessment and discuss with you your baby's well-being and demeanor. She will check your baby's sight by moving a rattle or other object across her field of vision and look for any signs of squinting.

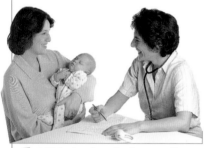

1 △ If she is asleep the doctor will wake her and assess how she responds to the stimulus of a new face, looking for a telltale smile or other sign.

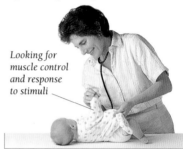

Looking for muscle control and response to stimuli

2 △ The doctor will then ask you to undress your baby to observe her muscle tone and to see how she moves her limbs.

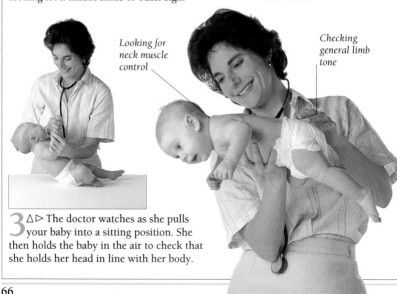

Looking for neck muscle control

Checking general limb tone

3 △▷ The doctor watches as she pulls your baby into a sitting position. She then holds the baby in the air to check that she holds her head in line with her body.

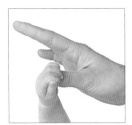

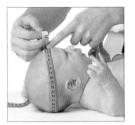

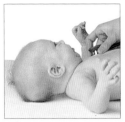

4 △ She then checks baby's grasp reflex by putting a finger into the baby's palm. This will have faded by six weeks.

5 △ Her head is measured to check for growth; a normal measurement is in the range of 15 in (38 cm).

6 △ The doctor listens to baby's heartbeat with a stethoscope. About 120 beats per minute is normal for the first year.

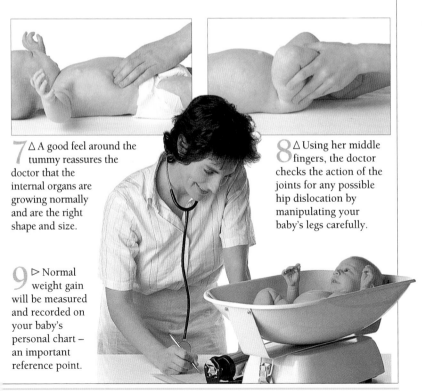

7 △ A good feel around the tummy reassures the doctor that the internal organs are growing normally and are the right shape and size.

8 △ Using her middle fingers, the doctor checks the action of the joints for any possible hip dislocation by manipulating your baby's legs carefully.

9 ▷ Normal weight gain will be measured and recorded on your baby's personal chart – an important reference point.

99 PREPARING FOR YOUR NEWBORN

Nothing can really prepare for the reality of having a new baby, especially a first child. The first weeks seem like a chaotic whirlwind as you and your partner go through a gamut of new experiences and adapt to being a family. But there are myriad baby items designed to make day-to-day living at home easier: you can borrow many of these from family or friends or buy them new or secondhand.

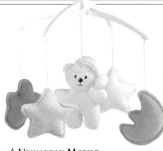

△ UPWARDLY MOBILE
With a new baby lying on his back for such long periods, a mobile above is ideal for eye stimulation.

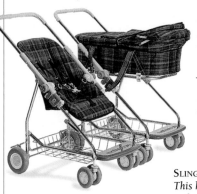

◁ BABY CARRIAGE
For the first three months your baby has to be able to lie flat so you should have a carriage. A stroller is for an older baby.

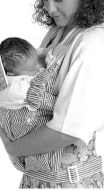

SLING APPEAL ▷
This keeps baby safe and secure while leaving your arms free. Great for indoor use or outdoor walking.

BATHTIME ESSENTIALS ▽
Make sure you have a large soft towel, baby bath, cotton balls, baby bath oil, and a washcloth or sponge.

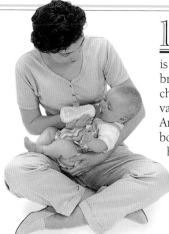

100 BREAST OR BOTTLE?

Breast is best for your baby: there is no substitute for the colostrum that your breasts produce in the first few days after childbirth. It will provide your baby with valuable antibodies to help fight infection. And, while you can switch from breast- to bottle-feeding, you cannot switch from bottle back to breast, because without the stimulation of your baby sucking, your breasts stop producing milk.

FEEL HAPPY WITH YOUR CHOICE
Feeling your baby will be no pleasure if you breast-feed from a sense of duty or bottle-feed with a sense of guilt.

101 BECOMING A FAMILY

Overwhelming pride, joy, round-the-clock exhaustion, responsibility for a tiny new person, the end of carefree life? These are just some of the emotions parenthood evokes. Often it is the father who is most shell-shocked in the days immediately after the birth, and he needs your support as much as you need his. Let him share in the care of your baby. Allow your confidence to grow.

PARTNER CHANGES
No longer just your lover, he's a companion and ally as a parent. Encourage him to be involved and active in child care.

A LEARNING CURVE
Looking after a baby requires your warmth, responsiveness, and attention. Some emotions are instinctive, some have to be learned.

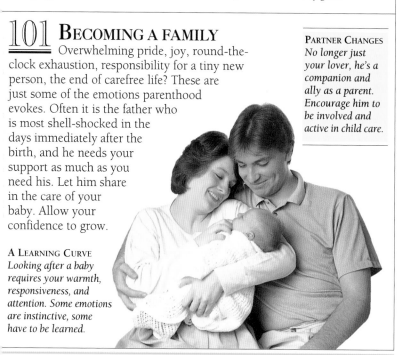

INDEX

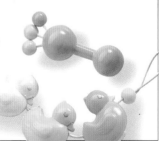

ACKNOWLEDGMENTS

Dorling Kindersley would like to thank Hilary Bird for compiling the index, Anne Crane for proofreading, Lesley Malkin for editorial assistance, and Mark Bracey for computer assistance.

Photography

KEY: t *top*; b *bottom*; c *center*; l *left*; r *right*

Antonia Deutsch 6, 12 ,13, 15, 16, 17cr, 18cl, 20, 24, 25tl, 26tr, 27bl, br, 30, 44, 45, 46t, br, 47tr, 48, 49, 61cl; Sally and Richard Greenhill 36tr; The Hutchison Library/ Nancy Durell McKenna 34b; Dave King 5br, 22tr, 27tr, 28, 29, 63tr, 66, 67, 69br; Ranald Mackechnie 1, 2, 9cl, 23, 26bl, 56, 57, 60br, 64br, 65, 68, 71; Stephen Oliver 5bl; Susanna Price 25 bl, br, 53, 54, 55, 63br; Julia Selmes 3; Tony Stone Images/ David Sutherland 34t; Ron Sutherland 52; Ian Thompson 61cr

Illustrations

Annabel Milne 14, 22br, 58tr
Coral Mula 17cl, 20, 46cl, 51, 58bl,br, 64 bl
Paul Williams 18br, Sharon Rudd 50tl

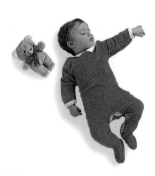